I0701591

HOW MUCH PROTEIN DO YOU ACTUALLY NEED

PROTEIN GUIDE FOR ALL

KATE .P

Contents

CHAPTER ONE

INTRODUCTION

Protein is a necessary macronutrient that is vital for many body processes, such as immune system function, muscular growth, and repair. Despite its significance, there is frequently misunderstanding about the amount of protein that a person should eat. Knowing how much protein you need will help you reach your fitness and general health objectives.

We'll explore the science underlying protein requirements, variables impacting personal needs, and useful tactics for achieving your protein intake targets in this guide. Knowing what amount of protein you need is essential to reaching your goals, whether you're a bodybuilder trying to gain muscle, a person trying to maintain a healthy weight, or someone just interested in improving your nutrition. In order to support your health and performance, let's examine how much protein you actually need and how to make sure you're receiving enough.

The necessity of protein in the diet

It is impossible to exaggerate the significance of protein in the diet because it is essential for so many aspects of general health and wellbeing. Here are several main justifications for why protein is necessary:

Building blocks of muscles, protein is necessary for the development, maintenance, and repair of muscles. Getting enough protein in your diet helps your muscles recover after a workout and keeps them from losing mass as you age or reduce your calorie intake.

Promotes Metabolism: Protein requires more energy to digest and metabolize than fats or carbs due to its increased thermic impact. This may facilitate weight control and fat loss by increasing metabolism and calorie expenditure.

Enhances Satiety: Foods high in protein are more filling than those high in fats or carbohydrates, which can help curb cravings and enhance appetite control. Goals for weight control can be supported and overeating can be avoided by including protein in meals and snacks.

Preserves Bone Health: Osteoporosis can be avoided and bone health can be preserved with the help of protein. It contributes to overall bone strength and density by giving bone tissue the building blocks it needs and by enhancing calcium absorption.

Supports Immune Function: Proteins make up a large number of immune system components, such as immune cells and antibodies. Eating enough protein strengthens the immune system and aids the body's defense against diseases and infections.

Aids in Hormone Production: Protein is necessary for the synthesis of hormones, enzymes, and neurotransmitters, which control a number of bodily physiological functions. A sufficient amount of protein is required for overall health and hormone balance.

Offers Vital Nutrients: Foods high in protein frequently include other vital nutrients including vitamins, minerals, and good fats. You can make sure you're getting the nutrients you need by include a range of protein sources in your diet.

Encourages Wound Healing: Tissue repair and wound healing depend on protein. Sufficient consumption of protein is imperative to bolster the body's capacity to mend impaired tissues and recuperate following trauma or operations.

Preserves Lean Body Mass: When cutting calories or losing weight, consuming adequate protein helps maintain lean body mass. Maintaining metabolic health, averting muscle loss, and encouraging long-term weight management all depend on this.

Helps Control Blood Sugar: Compared to carbs, diets high in protein have less of an effect on blood sugar levels. Protein can lower the risk of insulin resistance and type 2 diabetes while stabilizing blood sugar levels during meals and snacks.

All things considered, protein is a necessary ingredient that supports many bodily processes, including immune system function, hormone production, muscle health, and metabolism. It is essential to consume enough protein in your diet in order to maximize your performance, general well-being, and health.

It's critical to comprehend protein requirements if you want to meet your dietary needs, maintain muscle growth, and maximize your health. Your body requires different amounts of protein depending on your age, gender, exercise level, muscle mass, and general health objectives. This is an explanation of how to figure out how much protein you need:

Determine Protein Requirements Based on Body Weight: Using body weight as a starting point is a popular way to determine protein requirements.

Adults should consume 0.8 grams of protein per kilogram of body weight each day, according to the Recommended Dietary Allowance (RDA). Individual protein requirements, however, could change based on things like muscle mass and activity level.

Take Your Activity Level Into Account: You might require more protein to assist muscle growth and repair if you often exercise or are physically active. Protein intakes should be higher for athletes and others who train hard; they should be between 1.2 and 2.2 grams per kilogram of body weight per day.

Analyze Muscle Mass: To support muscle protein synthesis, people with higher muscle mass or those looking to gain muscle may find that eating more protein is beneficial. Maximum muscle protein synthesis and muscle growth may be achieved by consuming 1.6 to 2.2 grams of protein per kilogram of body weight each day, according to research.

Think About Your Health Objectives: Depending on your health objectives such as weight loss, weight maintenance, or muscle growth your protein requirements may change. Increased protein consumption during calorie restriction can increase satiety, maintain lean body mass, and encourage fat loss. Protein consumption at the higher end of the suggested range may be beneficial for those looking to maintain or reduce weight.

Spread Protein Intake Throughout the Day: Rather of ingesting significant amounts of protein at one meal, it's vital to divide protein intake evenly throughout the day to increase muscle protein synthesis and improve nutrient utilization. For the purpose of promoting muscle health and fullness, try to include a source of protein with every meal and snack.

Select High-Quality Protein Sources: Make an effort to incorporate a range of high-quality protein sources, such as dairy products, lean meats, chicken, fish, eggs, and tofu, into your diet. These foods supply the vital nutrients and amino acids required for optimum health and muscle growth.

Keep an eye on how your body reacts to the amount of protein you're currently consuming, and make any necessary adjustments based on your goals, level of exercise, and general wellbeing. Tracking alterations in your satiety, energy, strength, and muscle mass will help you make gradual modifications to your protein consumption.

To promote optimal health and performance, you can assess your specific protein requirements and adjust your diet by taking into account parameters like body weight, activity level, muscle mass, and health goals. Personalized advice on fulfilling your protein requirements and reaching your dietary objectives can also be obtained by speaking with a certified dietitian or other nutrition specialist.

Protein Recommended Daily Allowance (RDA)

Health authorities developed the Recommended Dietary Allowance (RDA) for protein as a guideline to give people the quantity of protein required to meet basic nutritional needs and maintain overall health. The RDA for protein is different for each age group, gender, and stage of life. The general RDAs for protein are as follows:

Adults: The recommended daily allowance (RDA) for protein in a healthy adult is 0.8 grams per kilogram of body weight. This indicates that in order to achieve their nutritional needs, an average inactive adult should try to ingest about 0.8 grams of protein per kilogram of body weight each day.

Women who are pregnant or nursing: To support the growth and development of the fetus and newborn, women's needs for protein rise during pregnancy and lactation. The recommended daily allowance (RDA) for protein during pregnancy is 1.1–1.3 grams per kilogram of body weight. The recommended daily allowance (RDA) for protein in lactating mothers is between 1.1 and 1.3 grams per kilogram of body weight.

Infants and Children: In order to sustain their rapid growth and development, infants and children have increased protein needs.

Depending on age, the recommended daily allowance (RDA) for protein in babies is 1.5 to 2.2 grams per kilogram of body weight. The recommended daily allowance (RDA) for children is 1.05 grams per kilogram of body weight for those aged 1 to 3, and 0.95 to 0.85 grams per kilogram of body weight per day for those aged 4 to 18.

Older persons: To maintain muscle mass and fend off age-related muscle loss (sarcopenia), older persons may require a somewhat higher protein intake. While most older persons still consume 0.8 grams of protein per kilogram of body weight per day as recommended by the RDA, some evidence indicates that older adults, especially those who are physically active or at risk of muscle loss, may benefit from larger protein intakes.

The Recommended Daily Allowance (RDA) for protein is a broad recommendation that might not take into consideration individual differences in activity level, muscle mass, metabolic rate, and state of health. Protein intakes may need to be increased for athletes, people with specific health goals, and people who participate in rigorous physical activity. Seeking advice from a qualified dietician or other healthcare professional might yield tailored suggestions based on unique circumstances and objectives.

Finding Your Protein Requirements

You must take into account a number of criteria when calculating your protein needs, including your age, gender, body weight, degree of exercise, and health objectives. This is a step-by-step strategy to help you figure out how much protein you need:

Determine Your Current Body Weight in Kilograms (kg) to begin the assessment of your weight. By dividing your weight in pounds by 2.20462, you may convert your weight from pounds to kilograms. If you weigh 150 pounds, for instance, your weight in kilograms would be about equal to 68 kg ($150 \div 2.20462 = 68$).

Think About Your Activity Level: A major factor in evaluating your protein requirements is your level of activity. In comparison to someone who is very active or participating in severe physical activity, such as strength training or endurance exercises, someone who is sedentary or lightly active may need less protein.

CHAPTER TWO

Determine Your Protein Needs Depending on Your Activity Level:

Sedentary/Lightly Active: To calculate your daily protein need, multiply your weight in kilograms by 0.8. For instance, your daily protein need would be roughly 54 grams if you weigh 68 kilograms (68 kg × 0.8 = 54).

Moderately Active: To calculate your daily protein need, multiply your weight in kilograms by 1.2 to 1.5. For moderate to intensive activity levels, choose a lower multiplier (e.g., 1.2) and a higher multiplier (e.g., 1.5). For instance, your daily protein needs could be between 82 and 102 grams if you weigh 68 kilograms and engage in moderate physical activity (68 kg × 1.2 = 82; 68 kg × 1.5 = 102).

Highly Active/Athletes: To calculate your daily protein requirement, multiply your weight in kilograms by 1.5 to 2.2. For endurance athletes, use a lower multiplier (e.g., 1.5) and for strength athletes or those doing a lot of resistance training, a larger multiplier (e.g., 2.2). For instance, your daily protein needs could be between 102 and 150 grams if you weigh 68 kilograms and are very active (68 kg × 1.5 = 102; 68 kg × 2.2 = 150).

Ajust for Particular Health Goals: Take into account any particular health objectives you may have, such as gaining muscle mass, decreasing weight, or healing from an injury. Higher protein intakes may help people gain muscle or recuperate from strenuous activity, whereas moderate protein intakes may help people lose weight by promoting satiety and maintaining muscle mass.

Protein Intake Should Be Spread Throughout the Day: To maximize muscle protein synthesis and promote general health and performance, divide your daily protein intake equally among meals and snacks.

Track Your Progress and Modify as Needed: Depending on changes in your activity level, muscle mass, and general health objectives, track your progress and modify your protein consumption as necessary. Seek advice from a qualified dietitian or other healthcare provider for recommendations that are tailored to your unique needs and situation.

You can make sure you're getting enough protein to support your overall health, fitness, and performance objectives by estimating your needs based on variables like body weight, activity level, and health goals. To maximize your nutrition and general well-being, keep in mind that each person may have different needs when it comes to protein. As such, it's critical to pay attention to your body and modify as necessary.

Quality and Sources of Protein

Protein sources differ greatly in terms of their nutritional makeup and quality. It's crucial to incorporate a range of protein sources in your meal plan to make sure you're getting all the nutrients and vital amino acids your body requires. The quality of a few popular protein sources is listed below:

Sources of Protein From Animals:

Meat: Lean cuts of lamb, chicken, hog, and cattle are great providers of premium protein. They are abundant in nutrients including iron, zinc, and vitamin B12 and supply all of the essential amino acids.

Fish and Seafood: High in protein and vital omega-3 fatty acids, fish and seafood include salmon, tuna, trout, shrimp, and shellfish. They're also rich in vitamins and minerals and low in saturated fat.

Eggs: Containing all nine necessary amino acids, eggs are a complete protein supply. They're also a great source of choline, selenium, and vitamins B12 and D.

Dairy Products: Milk, cheese, and yogurt are great providers of calcium, protein, and other vital elements. Reduce your intake of saturated fat by choosing dairy products that are low- or non-fat.

Sources of Plant-Based Protein:

Legumes: Pease, beans, lentils, and chickpeas are high in fiber, protein, and minerals. They are a heart-healthy protein option because they are also free of cholesterol and low in fat.

Soy Products: Complete protein sources made from soybeans include tempeh, tofu, edamame, and soy milk. They may be added to many different meals and are high in protein, fiber, and phytonutrients.

Nuts and Seeds: High in fiber, protein, and good fats are almonds, walnuts, peanuts, chia seeds, and hemp seeds. They're also a great source of antioxidants, minerals, and vitamins.

Quinoa: Quinoa is a whole grain free of gluten and a complete protein source because it has all nine necessary amino acids. It has a lot of fiber, vitamins, and minerals as well.

Sources of Processed Protein:

Protein Powders: Whey, casein, soy, pea, and rice protein powders are easy ways to enhance your consumption of protein, especially if you're an athlete or have higher protein requirements. Select premium protein powders with as little artificial additives and additional ingredients as possible.

Plant-Based Meat Substitutes: Tofu-based burgers, seitan, and plant-based protein patties are a few examples of the growing popularity of plant-based meat alternatives. While vegetarian and vegan diets might offer handy options, it's important to select items with little processing and extra substances.

Think at things like protein content, amino acid profile, nutrient density, and overall health impact when assessing protein sources. To make sure you're getting all the nutrients you need and having a varied, well-balanced diet, try to include a range of protein sources in your diet. Always prioritize whole, minimally processed meals, and seek individualized nutrition guidance from a qualified dietitian or other healthcare provider.

Required Protein for Various Objectives

Individual characteristics including age, gender, body weight, degree of activity, muscle mass, and particular health objectives can all affect one's protein requirements. Optimizing your protein consumption in accordance with your objectives is crucial for enhancing general wellbeing, performance, and health. The following lists the requirements for several types of protein:

Overall Well-Being and Upkeep:

The Recommended Dietary Allowance (RDA) for protein is 0.8 grams per kilogram of body weight per day for the majority of inactive or moderately active adults. This quantity is adequate to support general health and maintenance as well as basic nutritional needs.

Sarcopenia, or the age-related loss of muscle mass, may be avoided in older persons by gradually increasing their protein consumption, according to certain research.

Strength and Gained Muscle:

Higher protein consumption may help boost muscle protein synthesis and repair in those looking to gain muscle or strength. According to research, the best daily protein intakes for maximal muscle growth and recovery may be between 1.6 and 2.2 grams per kilogram of body weight.

Consuming a sufficient quantity of foods high in protein both prior to and following exercise is crucial for promoting muscle repair and recuperation.

Losing Fat and Weight:

During calorie restriction, protein is essential for maintaining lean body mass, fostering fat loss, and assisting with satiety. Increased protein consumption can aid in boosting fat loss by preventing muscle loss, increasing feelings of fullness, and reducing hunger.

Studies indicate that consuming 1.2 to 1.6 grams of protein per kilogram of body weight per day may help reduce body fat and promote weight loss, particularly when paired with consistent activity and a well-balanced diet.

Exercise and Performance for Endurance:

In order to assist muscle repair and recovery, endurance athletes may require a somewhat higher amount of protein, particularly during times of intense training or competition. For endurance activity, protein intakes between 1.2 and 1.4 grams per kilogram of body weight per day may be adequate to fulfill the increased demands.

Consuming lipids and carbohydrates is also necessary to maximize performance and supply energy for endurance exercises.

Recuperation following Surgery or Injury:

Protein requirements may rise after surgery or an accident to aid in wound healing, tissue repair, and recuperation. Increased protein consumption can aid in accelerating healing, preventing muscle loss, and enhancing general recuperation.

For individualized advice based on the kind and extent of the surgery or injury, speak with a qualified dietitian or healthcare provider.

It's crucial to remember that each person's requirements for protein may differ depending on a number of variables, including degree of exercise, muscle mass, metabolic rate, and general health. Keeping an eye on changes in your strength, energy, body composition, and general well-being can help you make gradual modifications to your protein consumption. Seek advice from a qualified dietitian or other healthcare provider for recommendations that are tailored to your individual needs and objectives.

Indications of Not Getting Enough Protein

A lack of protein can be indicated by a number of symptoms that can arise from an inadequate consumption. Many biological processes, such as immune system function, hormone generation, muscle growth and repair, and nutrient delivery, depend on protein. The following are warning indicators of low protein consumption to be aware of:

Protein is essential for preserving muscular mass and strength in the event of muscle loss or weakness. Weakness, diminished muscular tone, and muscle loss can result from consuming insufficient amounts of protein. You might experience diminished strength, a reduction in physical performance, or trouble doing daily duties.

Post-exercise Muscle Repair and Recovery: Protein is essential for muscle repair and recovery. Reduced exercise performance, prolonged muscular pain, and delayed recovery from exercises can all be caused by an inadequate protein consumption. It's possible that you're stuck at a certain level in your training or that it takes you longer to recuperate between sessions.

Fatigue and Weakness: Protein contributes to the synthesis of energy and aids in blood sugar regulation. An inadequate protein intake can cause sluggishness, weakness, and weariness. You can struggle to focus and concentrate during the day, or you might feel lethargic most of the time.

Protein is necessary for sustaining strong hair follicles and encouraging hair growth in cases of hair loss or thinning. A diet low in protein can cause thinning, hair loss, or textural changes in the hair. With time, you can observe a decrease in hair volume, more hair breakage, or greater shedding.

Protein can strengthen and encourage healthy nail growth in those with brittle nails. Slow nail development, ridges, and brittle nails might result from a low protein diet. Your nails may break easily, split easily, or peel easily, which could be a sign of a protein shortage.

Inadequate Wound Healing: Tissue repair and wound healing depend on protein. Insufficient consumption of protein can hinder the body's capacity to mend cuts, wounds, or injuries. You can encounter poor scar formation, accelerated infection susceptibility, or delayed wound healing.

Reduced immunological Response: Protein is essential for boosting immunological response and generating antibodies that aid in infection defense. A low protein diet can impair immunity, increasing your risk of infections, diseases, and immune-related conditions.

Protein helps keep the body's fluid balance and reduces excessive fluid retention, which can lead to edema or swelling. Insufficient consumption of protein can cause fluid imbalances, which can cause edema, or swelling, in the hands, feet, ankles, or abdomen. In certain locations, especially after extended durations of sitting or standing, you may detect puffiness or bloating.

You should evaluate your protein intake and make the required changes if you encounter any of these indications or symptoms to make sure you're getting the nutrients you need. Lean meats, chicken, fish, eggs, dairy products, legumes, nuts, and seeds are just a few examples of foods high in protein that you may include in your diet to help prevent protein deficits and promote general health and wellbeing. For tailored advice and recommendations, speak with a qualified dietitian or other healthcare expert if you have questions about your protein consumption or if your symptoms are not going away.

Dangers of Consuming Too Much Protein

Although getting enough protein is necessary for good health, getting too much of it can have negative consequences on the body. The following are some dangers connected to consuming too much protein:

Kidney strain: Because the kidneys are in charge of filtering waste materials produced by protein metabolism, a high protein diet may impose undue load on them. Eating too much protein can put more strain on the kidneys, which could damage them or make pre-existing kidney issues worse.

Dehydration: Water is needed for the metabolism of protein, and consuming too much protein might cause an increase in fluid loss through urine. Insufficient water intake can lead to electrolyte imbalances, dehydration, and possible kidney problems. To stay hydrated when eating a high-protein diet, it's critical to drink lots of water.

Digestive Problems: Eating a lot of protein, particularly animal protein, can cause digestive problems like diarrhea, bloating, and constipation. This is because protein sources derived from animals are frequently associated with high fat and low fiber contents.

Imbalances in Nutrients: If you eat a lot of meals high in protein, you could not be getting enough of other important nutrients including fats, carbohydrates, vitamins, and minerals. For overall health and nutritional balance, a diet rich in a variety of nutrient-dense foods is essential.

Increased Risk of Chronic Diseases: According to certain research, consuming too much protein, especially from animal sources, may put one at higher risk of developing certain chronic conditions like cancer, osteoporosis, and heart disease.

CHAPTER THREE

Diets heavy in protein might include higher levels of cholesterol and saturated fats, which can be harmful to heart health.

Weight Gain: Overindulging in protein can result in an overabundance of calories consumed, which over time may cause weight gain. Even though protein fills you up, eating more than your body requires can still lead to an excessive intake of calories, particularly if you combine it with high-calorie meals or drinks.

Nutritional Deficiencies: Over-reliance on high-protein foods or supplements might result in a lack of other vital elements that are present in whole grains, fruits, vegetables, and other dietary categories. To ensure that you get all the nutrients you need, you must eat a varied, balanced diet.

Bone Health: According to certain research, diets high in protein, especially animal protein, may have detrimental effects on bone health as well as increased excretion of calcium. To properly grasp the connection between protein consumption and bone health, more research is necessary.

It's crucial to remember that the dangers of consuming too much protein can differ based on personal characteristics like age, gender, degree of exercise, and general health. Moderate protein consumption within suggested ranges is unlikely to be harmful for the majority of healthy persons. However, before making big adjustments to their protein consumption, people with specific medical illnesses or kidney problems should speak with a healthcare provider. To support general health and well-being, it is always preferable to aim for a balanced diet that contains a variety of nutrient-dense foods.

Adapting Protein Consumption to Personal Requirements

For the purpose of supporting particular objectives, addressing special dietary demands, and maximizing health, protein consumption must be customized to meet individual needs. Here's how to adjust your protein consumption according to different factors:

Analyze Your Objectives: Establish your fitness and health objectives, including weight loss, muscular growth, enhanced athletic performance, and overall health preservation. Your objectives will affect your protein requirements and assist you in figuring out the right amount to consume.

Examine Your Activity Level: Pay attention to how much you exercise and how active you are each day. Higher protein consumption may be necessary for people who exercise frequently or are more physically active in order to assist muscle recovery and repair.

Determine Your Protein Requirements: Based on variables including body weight, degree of exercise, and particular objectives, determine your protein requirements using formulas or guidelines. The Recommended Dietary Allowance (RDA) is a good place to start; then, based on your unique situation, adapt as necessary.

Factor in Muscle Mass: larger protein intakes may be necessary to promote muscle growth and maintenance if you routinely perform strength training or have a larger muscle mass. Take into account your lean body mass and modify your protein consumption accordingly.

Evaluate Your Dietary Preferences and Restrictions: Consider any dietary preferences, limitations, or intolerances you may have, like veganism, vegetarianism, or dietary sensitivity to certain foods. Select protein sources that provide all of the required amino acids and fit your dietary choices.

Spread Your Protein Intake Throughout the Day: Try to split up your daily protein consumption equally between meals and snacks. Maximizing muscle protein synthesis and promoting satiety can be achieved by including protein in each meal.

Select High-Quality Protein Sources: Make an effort to incorporate lean meats, chicken, fish, eggs, dairy products, legumes, nuts, seeds, and tofu into your diet. These foods supply the vital nutrients and amino acids required for optimum health and function.

Track Your Development: Observe how your body reacts to the amount of protein you are currently consuming and make any necessary adjustments. To find out if your protein consumption is sufficient for your needs, track changes in your energy levels, muscle mass, strength, recuperation, and general well-being.

Speak with a Professional: You should think about speaking with a registered dietitian, nutritionist, or other healthcare provider if you have any specific health issues, nutritional concerns, or performance goals. They can offer tailored advice and suggestions depending on your particular requirements and situation.

You may meet your dietary requirements, support your fitness and health objectives, and enhance your general well-being by adjusting your protein intake to your specific needs. Keep in mind that each person may have different demands when it comes to protein, so it's important to pay attention to your body and modify as necessary to get the best outcomes.

Summary

To sum up, figuring out how much protein you truly need is a customized procedure that considers a number of variables, including your age, gender, body weight, degree of exercise, muscle mass, and specific health objectives. Although the Recommended Dietary Allowance (RDA) offers a broad recommendation for protein intake, several factors may cause individual needs to differ.

Achieving particular exercise objectives, sustaining general health, and promoting muscle growth and repair all depend on meeting your demands for protein. Tailoring your protein intake to meet your specific needs is essential, regardless of your goals maintaining a healthy lifestyle, gaining muscle mass, decreasing body fat, or improving sports performance.

You may adjust your diet to make sure you're receiving enough protein to support your needs by evaluating your goals, taking into account your activity level, estimating your protein requirements, and selecting high-quality protein sources. In order to maximize your protein consumption and general nutrition, it's also critical to track your progress, pay attention to your body, and make any necessary adjustments.

Speaking with a qualified dietician or other healthcare provider can offer tailored advice and suggestions based on your unique situation and objectives. You can support your health, improve your performance, and reach your goals with a balanced approach to protein intake and general nutrition.

THE END

www.ingramcontent.com/pod-product-compliance
Lightning Source LLC
Chambersburg PA
CBHW051922250726
48659CB00002B/785